# Dyslexia and the Bilingual Learner

*Assessing and Teaching Adults and Young People who Speak English as an Additional Language*

D1608642

# Contents

# Introduction

## Why the book was written

"How can I tell if my student's difficulties are due to learning English or because she is dyslexic?" is a common question among tutors teaching English to speakers of other languages and among dyslexia support tutors working with bilingual students.

Literature on the subject is sparse; not least because of the complexities of bi and multilingualism (for instance the age the person started learning English, the amount of schooling in the first or indeed second or third languages and the number of languages spoken and when they were learned) but also because of the subtle nature of dyslexia as a syndrome and the variation in the pattern of features displayed.

The ESOL and Dyslexia Working Party was set up to look into this question, drawing on the experience of a number of tutors experienced in assessing and teaching dyslexic students, ESOL students and bilingual dyslexic students. We met on a regular basis, over a period of three academic years.

As we explored, we became aware that assessment was not the only issue; the dyslexic learning style had implications for teaching dyslexic students in ESOL classes or for providing language support. In addition, the dyslexia support teacher needed to know something of the cultural and linguistic factors which might affect the bilingual dyslexic student's learning.

## About the book

This book addresses itself to ESOL and language support tutors who wish to learn something about dyslexia and how it may affect their students, and dyslexia support tutors who are concerned about diagnosing and teaching bilingual learners.

ESOL and language support tutors will find **Section 1** and **Section 3** particularly helpful, while tutors involved in dyslexia diagnosis and support should read **Section 2** and **Section 3**.

Throughout we have used the term 'bilingual' to refer to students who regularly use two or more languages in their daily lives. The term does not imply a particular level of proficiency in those languages. We are aware that many people speak more than two languages on a regular basis and are, in fact, multilingual.

We have used 'he' and 'she', 'his' and 'her' interchangeably throughout the book to refer to dyslexic learners of both sexes. Similarly we have used either 'tutor' or 'teacher' to refer to anyone who teaches.

Dyslexia and the Bilingual Learner; *Assessing and Teaching Adults and Young People who Speak English as an Additional Language*

*1*

# What is dyslexia?

At a recent conference, a speaker said she had discovered 82 different definitions of dyslexia! While arriving at a consensus definition is clearly difficult, we can say that it is a condition which affects a person's language processing abilities and may cause difficulties with aspects of written language, for instance reading, spelling and handwriting, and may affect some areas of speech, for instance word retrieval and pronunciation of particular sounds. It may affect ability to sequence and order material which affects study skills such as planning and essay or assignment writing. It usually affects short-term memory and ability to memorise by rote, common examples include difficulty in remembering the alphabet and tables. Dyslexic people may also have difficulties with directions and time, and confusion between right and left.

For language teachers the definitions that have the most resonance are the ones that look at dyslexia as a language processing difficulty, for instance the following one by Vellutino in 1987:

> "...its roots in a dysfunction during storage and retrieval of linguistic information; phonological-coding deficits (inability to represent and access the sound of a word); deficient phonemic segmentation (inability to break words into component sounds); poor vocabulary development and trouble discriminating grammatical and syntactic differences among words and sentences."[1]

## Language learning difficulties for dyslexic learners

Hannah Klein, (1985)[2] has written about how children with poor reading and writing skills are often attempting to superimpose these skills onto a poor oral base, and she hypothesises that it is for this reason that they fail to learn the skills. She gives examples of dyslexic children who were referred to her for poor literacy but who, like other dyslexic children, scored high on intelligence tests. When she tested them orally she found that some also had poor short term verbal memories, others scored low on tests of receptive and productive vocabulary, and yet others could not master complex linguistic structures (such as the passive) or did not understand puns, idioms, analogies or abstract vocabulary. If these are the problems in the children's first language, it is to be expected that the children would have considerable difficulty in learning an additional language.

Research done in the United States shows that "poor foreign language learners have less developed native language skills, particularly at the phonological/orthographic levels." (Ganschow and Sparks, 1995 - see Useful Books and Resources). Thus, some of the difficulties faced by dyslexic learners

Dyslexia and the Bilingual Learner; *Assessing and Teaching Adults and Young People who Speak English as an Additional Language*

3

when learning to read and write their first language will also affect their ability to learn a subsequent language.

If we take the approach that dyslexia is a difficulty in processing language, then this can be broken down further into difficulties with auditory, visual and motor processing. Dyslexic people may experience difficulties in one or more of these three areas, though usually one predominates.

Probably the most significant area for language learners is difficulty with auditory processing. Dyslexic learners with problems in this area are likely to have a poor auditory memory, difficulty discriminating sounds, and difficulty breaking down sounds into syllables or phonemes. They will have a problem with sound/symbol correspondence which will result in bizarre spelling and problems decoding unfamiliar words when reading. They may have difficulties retrieving vocabulary (i.e. finding the 'right' word), and in reproducing sounds, particularly pronouncing multisyllable words. These are all problems that can affect dyslexic learners in their first language. When these problems transfer into learning subsequent languages, it can easily be imagined that they will bring substantial added difficulties.

People with visual processing difficulties may have problems getting print to stabilise (complaining that it blurs, or jumps around). They may have difficulties in ordering and sequencing, which for language learners may translate into difficulty with sentence structure and word order. They have poor visual memories, meaning that they have a small sight vocabulary and have to rely more on 'sounding out' when reading. This slows reading down, and delays engagement with meaning. Copying, from the board will prove very difficult, particularly if the script is new to the student, as the words need to be held in the short term visual memory before being transferred onto paper. Both sequencing and poor visual memory affect spelling, letters are often mis-sequenced and words spelt phonetically. This is a strategy which may have worked in the past if the language learner's first language is phonetically regular, but will not work with the English spelling system.

Motor processing difficulties affect handwriting, and in turn spelling, which is partly learnt and retained through the motor memory. People with motor processing difficulties have problems controlling the pen, producing even and tidy handwriting, and often find writing very tiring. This occurs in learners' first languages, and if the script of subsequent languages is different, then their problems will be exacerbated.

# Should I refer?

The ESOL or language support tutor may come across students in their classes for whom learning English seems particularly difficult. With these students it may not seem reasonable to attribute all their difficulties in acquiring written English language skills to the fact that they are learning another language. There may be features, for instance spelling errors, which do not fit expectations of similar speakers of that particular language, or the learner may show extreme discrepancies between oral and written English, even when his educational background has been taken into account, or he may seem to be bright and motivated yet make very slow progress. In some cases this may be due to dyslexia, and the tutor needs to know when a referral for a specialist assessment for dyslexia is appropriate.

Dyslexia is normally diagnosed by identifying characteristic features, as mentioned, and by significant discrepancies in a student's performance in a range of skills.

Common discrepancies will often be between oral and written language skills, between reading level and spelling/writing level, between level of understanding and written expression, between written work when there is plenty of time and work under timed conditions.

The checklist below is not exhaustive but seeks to set out possible difficulties students may have which may be caused by dyslexia.

Tutors will need to take into consideration other possible causes for students' difficulties in reading, writing, understanding and speaking English. For instance, the student may have had little or disrupted education, and/or may be confusing English with other languages he knows.

However, if a student is dyslexic, he will demonstrate difficulties in English *and in his other languages*. But the difficulties which show up may vary, depending on the nature of these languages. For example, a student with poor visual word recognition can use a phonic approach to reading in a phonically regular language such as Spanish and thus his visual problems may not be apparent. In addition, unpublished research by Lindsay Peer[3] shows that bilingual dyslexic learners may have relatively few difficulties with their first language, but that the increase on the memory load means that they have real problems acquiring a second.

Tutors should note that most students will not manifest *all* these problems, but it is important to look for *a pattern of difficulties* and sometimes the tutor may need to observe the student's learning over a period of time.

---

Dyslexia and the Bilingual Learner; *Assessing and Teaching Adults and Young People who Speak English as an Additional Language*

5

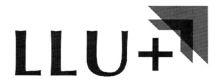

# A checklist for ESOL and language support tutors

**Tutors should consider the following questions:**

## 1.  Learning in the student's own language

- does the student have difficulties in learning to read, and problems with spelling or handwriting in any language?

- does the student have difficulties with 'finding the right word' in any language?

## 2.  What language problems would you expect?

- is there something that puzzles you about this student?

- is there an inexplicable lack of progress even after a period of time, with good tuition?

- does the student seem not to learn by 'ordinary' teaching methods? does the student demonstrate different kinds of difficulties to students of similar language backgrounds?

- does the student use bizarre spellings, not consistent with what you might expect from his language background?

- is there an unexpectedly wide discrepancy between writing and speech (even when educational background and difference of script are taken into account)?

- does the student's handwriting show the following features; irregularity of size, difficulty with control, messy, a lot of crossing out, a lack of progress in relation to other students of a similar language background?

- does the student have difficulty seeing mistakes, maybe writing the same word three different ways without noticing?

- does the student have persistent difficulty in remembering which letters represent which sounds (even when her own sound/symbol system has been taken into account)?

- is the student unable to recognise familiar words in print, even with reinforcement and repetition?

- does the student persistently mis-copy?

Dyslexia and the Bilingual Learner;  *Assessing and Teaching Adults and Young People who Speak English as an Additional Language*

7

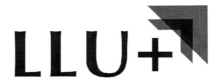

### 3.   Memory

- *does the student have a poor short term memory - for instance understands, but has a problem retaining information (a quick forgetter, rather than a slow learner)?*

- *does the student confuse or have difficulty remembering names, dates or facts (for instance, tables or new vocabulary)?*

- *does the student have particular difficulty in following language drills and remembering and repeating language patterns?*

### 4.   Sequencing and direction

- *does the student get letters or numbers out of order or back to front, for instance 26 for 62, 29 for 26?*

- *does the student experience left/right confusions?*

- *does the student have difficulty learning the alphabet or months of the year in sequence?*

- *does the student have problems following directions or verbal instructions in order?*

### 5.   Personal

- *does the student have 'good days' and 'bad days'?*

- *does the student feel frustrated by his inability to make progress and tendency to forget what he has learnt?*

- *does the student find it difficult to organise himself, work or time?*

**These factors are only indicators when there is a history of difficulties and they are persistent over a period of time.**

# Cultural and Linguistic Factors that may affect Diagnosis

When students speak, read and write other languages, features of these languages can influence the way they approach English. Tutors assessing bilingual students for dyslexia need to be aware of how these features could affect students' use of English, so that they do not confuse them with indicators for dyslexia.

In the last language census conducted in London (1987), over 170 languages were spoken by children in London schools. Surveys on this scale have not been done since, but it is likely that the number of languages has increased since then. It is not possible to describe all the features of all these languages, though some examples are given below. These have mostly been taken from *Learner English* (see **Useful Books and Resources**). Tutors can become familiar with features of the most common languages spoken in their colleges by talking to students, to tutors who share the students' languages, to ESOL and language tutors, and through works like *Learner English*.

## Phonology

Stress patterns may be different in different languages. For example, in Vietnamese only the first syllable is pronounced clearly and with stress. Additional syllables may sound indistinct to an English ear; therefore if a Vietnamese speaker uses the same strategy to decode English words, it may be that he/she recognises the second syllable but does not pronounce it as an English person would.

There are some sounds that we have in English that may not exist in students' own languages, or may be used inter-changeably. For instance, Spanish and most varieties of Catalan, only have one sound in the area of /b/ and /v/. Thus the student may appear to have difficulty in recognising the letter 'b' when in fact he is using the sound/symbol relationship from his own language.

## Spelling

If the student's own language is completely phonetic (for instance, Portuguese) and he is not used to writing in a language that is not phonetic, his visual memory may not be so well developed and he may falsely appear to have visual processing difficulties.

If the language does not contain consonant clusters within single syllables, such as Farsi, then students may put vowel sounds in-between consonant clusters for instance 'secool' for 'school'.

## Grammar

Differences in syntax and grammar can influence a student's ability to predict and make sense of texts when reading, or to write accurately in standard English.

The student's own language may have a different word order; for instance, in Arabic writing, the verb is placed first in the sentence and followed by the subject. There are no articles in many Eastern European languages, consequently students find it hard to use them in a consistent way.

Most languages have a different tense system. Some, for example Chinese, do not change the form of the verb and will use a word like 'yesterday' to support the past tense so that the sentence would translate as 'I go yesterday'.

## Handwriting

If students write in a different script, what may appear to be motor difficulties may be unfamiliarity with our script.

Forming letters and writing on the line may cause difficulties due to differences in students' own scripts. For example, Farsi is written in Arabic script and goes from right to left. Other languages, for instance Bengali, hang from the line rather than sit on the line.

The lack of written vowels in certain languages, such as Hebrew or Arabic means that students used to writing these languages may consistently omit vowels.

## Punctuation

Punctuation conventions vary in different languages. For instance, in Tigrinya, there are marks which look like our full stops after every word. Some languages, such as Thai, do not distinguish between upper and lower case. Thai words are not separated by spaces, and spaces are put in places where we would put punctuation, that is to indicate the end of a sentence. If students are transferring their punctuation conventions to English, they may miss out full stops or capital letters.

## Alphabet

A student's inability to remember the sound of a particular letter in English may appear to signal auditory processing difficulties, but in reality be as a result of differences in alphabets and the relationship of sound to symbol in her language. Particularly where students use the Roman script we expect them to be able to learn English with fewer problems but this process is not always so straightforward. Different languages that use the Roman Alphabet tend to have their own particular sound/symbol connections. For instance, some alphabets include completely different letters which do not exist in English script (for instance ß in the German alphabet) and some have the same symbol but have a different sound. for instance 'cc' in Italian sounds like our 'ch'. A script such as Cyrillic is particularly confusing. Some letters are the same as the Roman script, some are different. There are some letters that appear in the Roman script that are not in Cyrillic script and vice versa. For instance, the sound sh in English is represented by one symbol '[illegible]' in Cyrillic. Other letters, such as H appear in both but have different sounds in each ('H' in Cyrillic sounds like 'N' in English).

## Discourse

The organisation of ideas varies in different cultures and languages. In English, we tend to make the main point first and then give the details. However, in other cultures, for instance Japanese, it may be more common to start with what we would call the elaboration and conclude with the main point. Thus a student who appears to have problems organising ideas may just be organising them according to his discourse conventions.

## Vocabulary

The volume of unknown vocabulary may cause difficulties for the student. A student's comprehension of a reading passage may be seriously affected by her lack of knowledge of the vocabulary rather than an inability to engage with the meaning whilst reading or listening.

There may be words that are similar to a student's own language but can have a different meaning in English, For instance, in French '*sympathique*' does not mean '*sympathetic*', but '*pleasant*'.

It is important to check the student's understanding at all points in the interview.

## Culture

Students may have a different view of teachers in other cultures; students may not ask questions because they may feel that it is disrespectful, or may reply to questions giving answers that they feel the teacher wants to hear. This could affect the accuracy of information given in the interview.

If a student is often late, it may not be due to problems with the concept of time, or telling the time, but may be because time is viewed in a different way within his culture.

Many students from overseas have more problems in accepting the diagnosis of dyslexia. This is partly because of the higher profile dyslexia has had in this country in recent years and the greater understanding of the problems involved in comparison to that in their countries. Also culturally, it is not always appropriate to admit there is a problem. Extreme sensitivity needs to be used to ensure that the words like 'disability' are not used and that learning styles and strategies are emphasised.

NB Most of the above examples are taken from *Learner English; A Teacher's Guide to Interference and other Problems* (see list of **Useful Books and Resources.**)

# The Diagnostic Interview

## Guidelines for assessing bi/multilingual students who have had all or part of their education overseas

The interview format is adapted from the one described in *Diagnosing Dyslexia* (See **Useful Books and Resources**). It is designed to elicit factors in the history and learning experience of the student and to identify characteristics which would lead to a diagnosis of dyslexia. The whole diagnostic process consists of the diagnostic interview, and analyses of reading, writing and spelling.

In conducting the interview, the assessor must establish whether the difficulties encountered by the student are due to dyslexia, to a very disrupted education, to accident or serious illness, or to the fact that the student is learning in a second, third or even fourth language. It may be necessary to work with the student over a period of time to be sure of the diagnosis.

If the student does not speak enough English to fully understand or reply to the questions, an interpreter should be used. It is important that the student understands the purpose of the interview, and what dyslexia is. She should not look on the interview as a test which has to be passed.

The following guidelines for the diagnosis of bilingual students are to be used with the adapted **Diagnostic Interview Form,** and are additional to the general guidelines which can be found in Chapter 2 of *Diagnosing Dyslexia*. They are given to aid in interpreting the significance of linguistic and cultural factors for the dyslexia specialist. The **Diagnostic Interview Form** has been adapted to elicit these linguistic and cultural factors which may affect bilingual students' acquisition of English as well as to identify a pattern of difficulties indicating dyslexia.

## Language History

You need to find out what languages the student speaks, understands, reads and writes, and how these languages work, in order to try and establish whether the student is actually dyslexic or is merely transferring features of her language when she is using English.

An explanation of how phonology, orthography and grammatical structure in different languages can affect a learner's acquisition and use of English is given in **Cultural and Linguistic Factors that may Affect Diagnosis.**

You need to note students' level of understanding of English and their spoken English. For speaking skills you need to note their fluency, grammatical accuracy, wide use of vocabulary, and complexity of spoken sentence structure. For comprehension, you should comment on students' understanding of the interview questions, as well as the speed of English you had to use. Also comment on their understanding of specific vocabulary and structural items; for instance do they understand conditional sentences such as *"if I gave you a list of directions, could you follow it?"*. If their speaking and understanding of English is much higher than their level of reading and writing, this discrepancy may be a pointer to dyslexia. If their spoken English is also at quite a low level, and they do not read and write in their own language(s), then diagnosis will be much more difficult.

## Schooling - General

It is important to ask for specific information about schooling - how many schools the students attended, how many years they attended the different schools, the language of instruction in the different schools, the styles of learning (for instance, were they expected to do much free writing or was it mainly copying and multiple-choice questions). You need to ask the same questions for **all** the schools that the students attended, as often students will only give information that they think you will find important.

It is not possible to assume that the terms 'secondary' or 'primary' will mean the same in the students' country as it does here. You may need to check the dates and ages that students attended each particular school. Ages, however, may also be misleading, as it is common practice in many countries for students to repeat classes until they pass the end-of-year exams.

If a student has been to school in this country, it is important to find out when she arrived, how many years of schooling she did here, and whether or not she was given language support, either in the classroom or in withdrawal groups. A student would usually be expected to pick up basic oral communication skills after having been in school in this country for 1 - 2 years. However, literacy is a much more complex and more slowly acquired skill. If the student arrives in primary school, she can expect to get direct literacy tuition. However, if she arrives in secondary school, she may never be taught basic literacy skills and may have had to 'pick them up' within her mainstream subject classes. Tutors need to ask how much explicit literacy tuition the student has received, for instance was she ever taught the names of the letters, or the sound/symbol relationship?

Outside England, it is quite usual for students to speak one language at home, to learn in a second language at primary school and to be educated in a third when starting secondary or middle school. Refugees may have missed a lot of schooling, or attended very basic 'schools' in refugee camps, where the facilities were not available for reading books or writing.

In order to draw conclusions about the student's reasons for poor literacy skills, you need to find out:

- *was the student at school and learning to read in the crucial early years?*

- *did she first learn to read her own or a second language?*

Dyslexia and the Bilingual Learner; *Assessing and Teaching Adults and Young People who Speak English as an Additional Language*

*13*

- *did she fall behind at school at any time, compared to her peers with a similar background? Did she have to repeat any years, or fail end-of-year exams?*

- *did she have any difficulties reading and writing in her language which could not be explained by disrupted schooling?*

- *how many years of English schooling did she do, and how much explicit literacy teaching was there during that time?*

## Language/Listening Behaviours

Establish whether the student has trouble in her own language, as well as English with the following:

- *does she find it difficult to concentrate in class/'take in' what the lecturer/teacher is saying*

- *if she's with a group of friends can she 'keep up' with the flow of topics?*

- *can she manage tongue twisters? Ask her to tell you one in her language.*

- *does she have trouble 'finding the right word'?*

- *has she ever tried to listen to a lecture and take notes, and found this difficult? - Is this because of difficulties with spelling, with understanding the English, or with trying to listen and write at the same time?*

- *when learning English, did she find it difficult to listen, repeat and remember common phrases?*

If you give her multisyllabic words to say, take care that you do not give consonant clusters (these may not occur in her own language). Try -*anemone, philosophical, aluminium, culinary.*

## Reading

Questions here should be asked about students' own languages as well as English.

Responses in this section should be looked at in the context of the reading analysis which is also part of the whole diagnostic process.

## Writing and Spelling

Questions here should be asked about students' own languages as well as English.

Responses in this section should be looked at in the context of the writing and spelling error analyses, which are part of the whole diagnostic process.

## Maths

Take into account the amount of formal education the student has had before asking the questions about, for instance, long division, algebra. Some refugees may never have had the chance to learn formally.

## Memory

Ask the student what difficulties she has remembering in her own language as well as in English. For instance, does she find taking telephone messages difficult in any language? Does she often get the message wrong?

Sequences, for instance, numbers, months of the year etc. both forward and backward, can be repeated in the student's own language, with the use of an interpreter.

## Spatial/Temporal

Difficulties in reading a map may be due to a disrupted education - i.e. the student may never have been taught to read a map.

## Visual/Motor

Use your knowledge of the student's first language and differences in writing conventions when making your assessment of the student's handwriting (see **Cultural and Linguistic Factors that may affect diagnosis**).

# The Diagnostic Interview

The following form has been devised to elicit linguistic and cultural factors, which may affect bilingual students' acquisition of English as well as to identify a pattern of difficulties indicating dyslexic/specific learning difficulties. The accompanying guidelines are given to aid in interpreting the significance of linguistic and cultural factors for the dyslexia specialist.

Dyslexia and the Bilingual Learner; *Assessing and Teaching Adults and Young People who Speak English as an Additional Language*

15

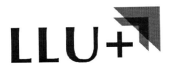

# DYSLEXIA

*Diagnostic Interview Form for bilingual students*

**Student should write name and address. Other questions to be completed by interviewer with the help of an interpreter if necessary.**

Student's Name: ...........................................................................................................

Date: ...........................................................................................................................

Address: ......................................................................................................................

.....................................................................................................................................

.....................................................................................................................................

Telephone: ...............................................  Age: (if relevant) ..............................

College/Institution: ....................................................................................................

Contact: ......................................................................................................................

Course/Work Info.: ...................................................................................................

**Considerations requested:**

☐ examinations ☐ extra time ☐ sympathetic consideration

☐ extra time in assignments ☐ other (specify)

.....................................................................................................................................

Other college/educational experiences since leaving school either in UK or another country:

Educational aims of student:

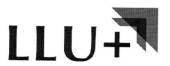

Attitude of teachers/success at school:


Attitude of student/self-assessment of difficulties:



Date of arrival in UK:.............................................................................................................

Age when arrived:.................................................................................................................

How long speaking English?.................................................................................................

## ● Language History

First language(s) (or language(s) spoken with family)

.................................................................................................................................................

.................................................................................................................................................

Languages taught in

.................................................................................................................................................

Languages spoken and understood (include level of English)

.................................................................................................................................................

.................................................................................................................................................

Languages read

.................................................................................................................................................

.................................................................................................................................................

| | | |
|---|---|---|
| Does writing go from left to right? | ☐ Yes | ☐ No |
| Is language phonetic? | ☐ Yes | ☐ No |
| Difficulty learning a second or third language? | ☐ Yes | ☐ No |

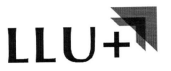

## ● Schooling - General

Ever been to school?  ☐ Yes  ☐ No

Years of schooling ..............................................................................................................

Schooling  (ages and languages used *for all schools*)

| SCHOOL | AGES | LANGUAGE USED |
|--------|------|---------------|
|        |      |               |
|        |      |               |
|        |      |               |
|        |      |               |
|        |      |               |
|        |      |               |
|        |      |               |

Amount of writing done at school

..............................................................................................................................

..............................................................................................................................

Multiple choice exercises?

..............................................................................................................................

..............................................................................................................................

Other kinds of writing (eg. was it writing where you were asked to give opinions?)

..............................................................................................................................

..............................................................................................................................

Types of reading done in school (eg. textbooks, handouts)

..............................................................................................................................

..............................................................................................................................

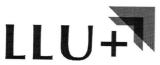

## ● Schooling - Primary (or equivalent)

Early problems learning to read and write

Received extra help/language support

Disruptions/missed school

## ● Schooling - Secondary (or equivalent)

Problems recognised by school

Received extra help

Fall behind at any stage of different schooling

Exams attempted (particularly English)

Exams passed/grades

Consideration given

## Any other comments/observations?

.............................................................................................................................

.............................................................................................................................

.............................................................................................................................

.............................................................................................................................

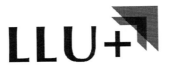

## ● Background/history

Ear infections/'glue ear' (early childhood)

Vision problems: squint/lazy eye/other

Motor-coordination problems (for instance
tying shoelaces/catching a ball or 'clumsy child' syndrome)

Speech or language difficulties/'late talker'
(in first language)

Other members of family have similar difficulties

Any serious health problems as a young child
(for instance respiratory, neurological)

Any serious accidents

### Any other comments/observations:

...................................................................................................................................................................

...................................................................................................................................................................

...................................................................................................................................................................

● ...................................................................................................................................................................

## Language/listening behaviours

Trouble listening (eg. in lectures, group discussions)

Trouble concentrating with background noise

Pronunciation difficulties? Especially with multi- syllabic words

Word retrieval problems

Problems listening and taking notes simultaneously

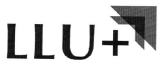

## ● Reading

**Approximate level:**    *in own language if literate:*

                                    *in English:*

Needs to re-read frequently

Comprehension difficulties

Word recognition problems

Decoding problems

Oral reading difficulties

Problems tracking print

Print 'dances', blurs or irritates eyes

## Approaches used by student:

........................................................................................................................

........................................................................................................................

........................................................................................................................

........................................................................................................................

## Any other comments/observations:

........................................................................................................................

........................................................................................................................

........................................................................................................................

........................................................................................................................

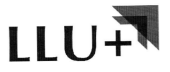

● **Writing and Spelling**

*With reference to own language as well as English if appropriate.*

**Approximate level:**    *in own language if literate:*

*in English:*

Difficulty getting ideas down on paper

Word retrieval problems

Problems with grammar and/or
sentence structure

Problems with structure and/or
punctuation

Problems with organisation and planning

**What planning strategies does student use:**

........................................................................................................................................................

........................................................................................................................................................

'Good' days and 'bad' days

Difficulties remembering what words
look like

Difficulties discriminating/'holding' sounds

Difficulties 'seeing' errors/proof-reading

**General spelling approaches used by student:**

........................................................................................................................................................

........................................................................................................................................................

**Any other comments/observations:**

........................................................................................................................................................

........................................................................................................................................................

........................................................................................................................................................

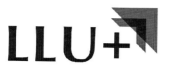

# ● Maths

Difficulties memorising times tables

Difficulties memorising basic number facts

General proficiency

Difficulties with long division/algebra, etc.

Other (specify)

.......................................................................................................................................................

**General approach:**

.......................................................................................................................................................

.......................................................................................................................................................

**Any other comments/observations:**

.......................................................................................................................................................

.......................................................................................................................................................

.......................................................................................................................................................

.......................................................................................................................................................

# ● Memorisational difficulties

Alphabet

Months or days forwards and backwards
(in own language as well as English)

Telephone numbers

Erratic memory

Names/dates/factual information

Difficulties remembering lists/sequence
of verbal instructions

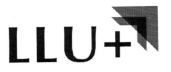

**Any other comments/observations:**

..................................................................................................................................

..................................................................................................................................

..................................................................................................................................

..................................................................................................................................

# Spatial/temporal/

Difficulties learning to tell time

Left/right confusion (eg. point to my
right ear with your left hand)

Gets lost easily

Map reading difficulties

Difficulties following oral directions

Mixing up bus numbers eg. 26 for 62,
29 for 26

Other (specify)

..................................................................................................................................

**Any other comments/observations:**

..................................................................................................................................

..................................................................................................................................

..................................................................................................................................

..................................................................................................................................

..................................................................................................................................

..................................................................................................................................

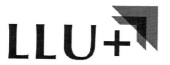

## Visual-motor

Copying difficulties

Letter/number reversals

Unusual paper position

Unusual pen grip

Left-handed

Use other hand for some tasks
If Yes, please state which ones

..................................................................................................................................................................

Difficulties controlling pen

Irregular or awkward letter construction

Problems with writing what is intended
/much crossing out, etc.

Hand gets tired after short period
of writing

*Ask student to write in own language.*

*Ask student to write something simple in English.*

*Compare handwriting in both languages.*

**Any other information/observations:**

..................................................................................................................................................................

..................................................................................................................................................................

..................................................................................................................................................................

..................................................................................................................................................................

# Additional diagnostic tests

It is difficult to assess students who are beginner readers and writers in English, and it may not be possible to come to a definite conclusion for the diagnosis. It may be necessary to observe the student over a period of time. You may still not reach a conclusion about whether or not he is dyslexic, but you should be able to make an assessment of his learning style, and evaluate what methods he finds work best for him. As we said earlier, it may be necessary to use an interpreter for students who are not fluent speakers of English, and it will certainly be necessary to ask questions about the student's reading and writing in his own language. If a student has never learnt to read and write in any language, and does not speak much English, it could be very difficult to do an accurate diagnosis.

The following additional tests may help you to make a diagnosis.

## Visual tests

- the student matches and draws shapes, symbols etc.

- the student picks out letters that look the same from a number of letters (See *Use your Eyes*, in **Useful Books and Resources**.)

## Sequencing and short term memory tests

The following can be done in English or the student's own language, using an interpreter.

- the student says the days of the week/months of the year forwards and/or backwards

- the student repeats lists of three to five numbers or letters that the tutor says (for instance *6-9-7* or *5-8-2-3*, starting off with three numbers, and going on to four if the student can repeat two lists in a row, and so on. The tutor must be sure to pause briefly between each number or letter. The average short term memory can contain seven items, plus or minus two, therefore if the student cannot remember three or four, there is some problem with her short term memory.

## Auditory tests

- non-words - the student repeats them after the tutor, (see *Diagnosing Dyslexia* for a list of these)

- odd one out - the student picks out the odd one from a group, for instance: cat, rat, fan, hat. These can be done with beginnings and middles as well as with endings

- rhyming - the student finds words that rhyme with words the tutor says, for instance: *jelly (telly)*

- number of syllables - the student identifies how many beats words have, for instance, circus, government, refugee, boat, etc.

## Blending and Segmenting

- the student is asked to identify a sound, for instance: the tutor says two words '*bead*' and '*bleed*', the student is asked to identify the extra sound

- the student is asked to take out the sound - for instance: the tutor says "*bleak*", and then asks the student to say it again without the '*l*' sound

- the student is asked to add sounds - for instance "*What word do you get if you add the sound 'p' to the word 'rinse'?*"

- student is asked to make words by putting two phonemes together - for instance "*What word do you get if you put the sounds 'sh' and 'oe' together?*"

- spoonerisms - the student makes spoonerisms, for instance: the tutor says "*John Lennon*", the student has to say "*Lohn Jennon*". This can be done with common two word phrases - for instance: '*car park*', '*coat hanger*', '*shoe box*', as well as with common names.

## Naming

- student is asked to name a particular letter (and identifies the sound it makes). This could be done in the student's own language, using an interpreter.

N.B.  These tests should always be done in conjunction with knowledge about the student's language(s). Only ask the student to identify sounds that exist in her own language(s).

# Reading Passages

## Notes to accompany the Reading Passages

The reading passages are to be used to conduct an analysis of the student's reading style and reading difficulties, using a miscue analysis and assessment of comprehension. For a detailed description of the methodology, see *Diagnosing Dyslexia*.

The passages have been chosen to reflect contexts and vocabulary that will be as familiar as possible to the student, so that difficulties in reading them are likely to reflect the student's reading process rather than difficulties with the English language. These factors, along with grammatical complexity have been taken into account when grading the passages. It is important to note that other readability tests, such as the Fogg index, do not take these factors into account. Thus a passage like 'Bob' in *Diagnosing Dyslexia* is graded as beginner level but may prove difficult for an ESOL student because of cultural context and idiomatic language.

No selections have been included for levels above intermediate, as students above this level will need to be able to read a variety of texts with a range of syntax, vocabulary and language usage. However, linguistic and cultural factors should always be taken into account when drawing conclusions from a reading analysis.

The beginner and elementary passages may be too short to generate the number of errors (approximately 25) to do an accurate miscue analysis. However, students at this level of English may find it extremely difficult to read for longer. If this is the case, you should use the reading passages to find out what you can about the student's reading style. For instance does she understand and retain what she reads? What strategies does she use with unfamiliar words? Is she a fluent or hesitant reader, does she omit words, repeat them, correct mistakes? You should then supplement the analysis with some of the techniques suggested in **Additional Diagnostic Tests**. It must be recognised that it may not be possible to make an accurate diagnosis with a student at this level of English, and you may need to work with the student and observe her over a period of time.

It is also useful, as with all students, to supplement the reading analysis with single-word and especially non-word tests (see *Diagnosing Dyslexia* for a list of single words. You should only ask the student to read words she is able to say and understand.)

It is always important to be clear about the reasons for a student's reading difficulties and to consider that they may be due to her lack of understanding of English.

When looking at miscues, take care to check whether the word the student cannot read is actually known to her, i.e. she can understand it when it is said to her. If she cannot understand it, her means of decoding unfamiliar words will also give you information about her strategies and her knowledge of English (for instance, can she 'sound out' phonetically?)

Also, take into account the student's level of spoken English when assessing the miscues. For instance, someone who is not familiar with English syntax will find it much more difficult to use syntax to predict. It does not, however, necessarily mean that the student does not understand the text she is reading.

The comprehension questions are given orally to the student without the student referring back to the passage. Thus memory of detail and sequence along with understanding of the gist can be assessed.

# The Cooking Pot

There was an old man called Nasreddin. He was a very funny man. One day he asked his friend if he could borrow a big cooking pot.

After a day had gone by Nasreddin gave his friend two cooking pots; one was slightly smaller than the other. The friend asked

"Why have you given me two cooking pots back?" Nasreddin replied to his friend: "The large cooking pot I borrowed from you had a baby." The friend was very pleased.

The next day Nasreddin went back to his friend and again he asked if he could borrow the cooking pot. The friend gave it to him.

After days went by Nasreddin did not return his friend's cooking pot. The friend asked Nasreddin:

"Why have you not returned my pot?" Nasreddin replied,

"I am afraid your cooking pot has died!" The friend asked

"How can a cooking pot die?" Nasreddin replied

"Well, you believed that your cooking pot had a baby so why don't you believe that your cooking pot has died?"

**beginner level**

1. Tell me in your own words what the story was about.

2. What did Nasreddin borrow in the first place?

3. What did Nasreddin give back?

4. How did he explain the difference?

5. What happened the second time?

6. Why was the friend unhappy?

7. Why do you think Nasreddin gave his friend two cooking pots at the beginning?

Story by Figen from Cyprus, from *Friends, Families and Folk Tales* (1997), London Language and Literacy Unit. Originally published in *Collections of Student Writing*, (1986) ESL Publishing Group, ILEA

# My poor friend Zehra

My friend's name was Zehra. She had blonde hair, brown eyes, fair skin. She was thin. She was a very kind and nice girl. I liked her because we were very good friends and we grew up together.

The day she died we went to a wedding party. We were playing, then we ran into the road. There was a car - it was coming very fast. She didn't see it. They were English soldiers, and they couldn't stop. They hit her and she died.

She was seven years old.

I still think about her, because we were best friends.

## beginner level

1. Tell me in your own words what the story was about.

2. Describe what Zehra looked like.

3. Why did Shoray like her?

4. What happened to Zehra?

5. How did it happen?

6. Where did they go that day?

7. How old was she?

8. Why did the accident happen?

Story by Shoray from Cyprus, from *Friends, Families and Folk Tales* (1997), London Language and Literacy Unit. Originally published in *Collections of Student Writing,* (1985) ESL Publishing Group, ILEA

# The Fox and The Stork

One day the fox met his friend the stork in the forest. He asked him for dinner. The fox promised to make a special dinner just for his friend. The stork accepted the invitation.

The next day the stork went to the fox's house. The fox put the special food (which was soup) in the saucer. The stork couldn't eat it and the fox ate all the soup. After a few hours the stork left.

The time came for the fox to go to the stork's house for dinner. The fox went but he couldn't eat because the stork put his food in a very tall, narrow jar. So the stork ate all the food, and after he finished he said to the fox, "Now it's my turn to laugh."

## beginner level

1. Tell me in your own words what the story was about.

2. Why did the fox invite the stork to dinner?

3. Why did the stork not eat the soup?

4. Why could the fox not eat the stork's dinner?

5. Can you explain why the stork said to the fox "Now it's my turn to laugh."

Adapted from a story by Stelios from Greece, from *Friends, Families and Folktales* (1997), London Language and Literacy Unit. Originally published in *Collections of Student Writing*, (1985) ESL Publishing Group, Language and Literacy Unit, ILEA.

# When I was a child

When I was a child we used to live in North Vietnam. My father used to work in a factory. My mother used to work in a big store. I remember I used to visit my mother's store to look at the things I liked but I didn't have any money to buy anything. My mother was very busy in the store.

When I was five I began to go to school, and every Monday to Friday I went to school to learn the Chinese language. When I was about twelve I started to help my mother look after my brother and sister.

## beginner level

1      Tell me in your own words what the story was about.

2.    Where did Phong live?

3.    Where did Phong's mother work?

4.    How old was Phong when she started school?

5.    Why did Phong visit the store?

6.    Why didn't she buy anything?

7.    What did Phong learn at school?

8.    How did she help her mother?

9.    What kind of life do you think Phong's mother had?

Story by Phong from Vietnam, from *Changes: Collections of Student Writing 3*, (1985) ESL Publishing Group, Language and Literacy Unit ILEA.

Dyslexia and the Bilingual Learner; *Assessing and Teaching Adults and Young People who Speak English as an Additional Language*

33

# My mother's life

I am writing about my mother's life, because it is the most remarkable life in my family.

My mother married when she was eleven years old. She had her first child when she was fourteen years of age. She was looking after the house and after her children at a time when she needed someone to look after her. But she did it perfectly.

She brought up all her children properly. She learnt to read and write at home because she hadn't had the chance to go to school at that time. She had a lot of knowledge that helped us when we were in the primary school. She helped us to read and to prepare our homework.

She suffered quite a lot from her big family, but at the end of the long journey she is very happy, because all her children have finished their higher education and got good jobs. This is what makes her very pleased and gives her comfort.

## elementary level

1.  Tell me in your own words what the story was about.

2.  When did the writer's mother get married?

3.  Does the writer think her mother was the right age to get married? If not, why not?

4.  Did she go to school?

5.  How did she help her children?

6.  Why is she so happy now?

7.  Do you think she has many children?

8.  What do you think the writer feels about her mother?

Story by Azhar from Iraq, from *Families and Friends, Collections of Student Writing 2*, (1985) ESL Publishing Group, Language and Literacy Unit, ILEA.

# A Terrible Journey

The journey took one month. We all paid two hundred pounds each for the fare, the same price for the children and adults. It was a terrible journey; nearly every day the sea was rough, and I'm not a very good sailor. Everybody was sick and unhappy. The women and children cried, as they were afraid of the sea and unhappy about leaving Vietnam.

The food we ate was cooked turnips and rice. The turnips were sliced and cooked in boiling water. The children and I slept most of the journey because we were so tired from being sick. Only the women and children were allowed in the lower part of the boat. It was too dangerous on the top deck as the waves were very high and came over the boat. The men had to stay on the top part of the boat.

On our boat were two captains. Now one is in Germany and the other is in Scotland. The captains were very mean with the food as they gave big portions to their families but very little to the other passengers. It was a terrible journey.

## elementary level

1. Tell me in your own words what the story was about.

2. How much was the fare for the journey?

3. How did they travel?

4. Why was the journey so difficult?

5. Where did the women and children sleep?

6. Why do you think the men had to stay on the top part of the boat?

7. What sort of food did the people eat on the boat?

8. Do you think they had enough food to eat?

9. Why do you think they were travelling on the boat?

Story by Tinh from Vietnam, from *Changes: Collections of Student Writing 3*, (1985) ESL Publishing Group, Language and Literacy Unit, ILEA.

# The Man and The Monkey

Long, long ago there was only one man in the world. One day the man went to the forest to cut wood for his fire.

When he got to the forest he took off his hat. He hung it on the branch of a tree and started to cut the wood. He cut enough wood to make a big bundle, put the bundle on his back and walked home.

He was nearly home when suddenly he remembered his hat. So he turned round and went back to the forest.

A monkey had been sitting in the tree watching the man. The monkey saw the hat and liked it. When the man left the forest, the little monkey jumped down from the tree, picked up the hat and put it on his head.

The man wanted his hat. When he got back to the forest he looked everywhere for it but he couldn't find it. He suddenly saw the monkey in the tree, with the hat on its head.

How was the man to get his hat? He couldn't catch the monkey. He thought for a long time. All the time the monkey watched him. Then the man had an idea. He pulled some hair from the top of his head, held it up in the air and threw it on the ground.

The monkey watched. Then the monkey pulled the hat from his head, held it up in the air and threw it on the ground. The man quickly picked it up, put it on his head and walked home.

**elementary level**

1. Tell me in your own words what the story was about

2. Why was the man in the forest?

3. What did he forget?

4. Tell us what the monkey did when the man went home.

5. Why did the man pull hair from the top of his head and throw it on the ground?

Story by Lan from Vietnam, from *Friends, Families and Folktales* (1997), London Language and Literacy Unit. Originally published in *Collections of Student Writing*, (1985) ESL Publishing Group, Language and Literacy Unit,

# The Bed

Is it difficult for you to get up in the morning? Do you sometimes oversleep? Are you often late for work or school? Yes? Then Hiro Sugiyama from Japan has a special bed for you. This bed will help you get up in the morning! Here is how it works.

The bed is connected to an alarm clock. First the alarm clock rings. You have a few minutes to wake up. Next, a tape recorder plays soft, pleasant sounds. A few minutes later the tape recorder plays something unpleasant, like loud music or someone shouting. Hiro's tape recorder first plays his girlfriend talking in a sweet voice. Then it plays his boss shouting "Get up immediately! You will be late for work!"

If you don't get up after that, you will be sorry. Inside the bed there is a mechanical 'foot' which kicks you in the head. After a few more minutes, the top of the bed rises slowly up into the air while the bottom of the bed gets lower and lower. Finally you will slide out of bed and onto the floor.

Unfortunately you cannot buy Hiro's bed in the shops. He only made one bed because he wanted to win a competition. Hiro won a prize for his bed and it has also solved his problem. Now he always gets up on time.

## post-elementary level

1.   Tell us in your own words about the story.

2.   What is special about Hiro's bed?

3.   How does the bed wake you up first?

4.   What are the nice sounds that Hiro hears?

5.   What are the nasty sounds?

6.   Why do the things that happen in Hiro's bed get more and more unpleasant?

7.   What other things does the bed do to make Hiro get up?

8.   Why can't you buy a bed like Hiro's?

Adapted from *More True Stories* by Sandra Heyer, Copyright © 1990. ISBN 0 8013 0223 4 Reprinted by permission of Addison Wesley Longman.

Dyslexia and the Bilingual Learner;  *Assessing and Teaching Adults and Young People who Speak English as an Additional Language*

37

# Money to Burn

Lillian Beard smiled as she worked. "Why are you so happy?" her friends asked her. "Yesterday I received a cheque for £462! This morning I went to the bank and cashed the cheque. I've got £462 in my pocket and I'm thinking about how I will spend it!"

After work Lillian went home. Her clothes were dirty so she took them off and put them in the washing machine. When she took them out, she suddenly remembered the money - she had left it in her pocket. She looked in her pocket. The money was still there but it was very wet. Lillian put the money on the kitchen table to dry.

After a few hours she felt the money. It was still very wet. "How can I dry this money?" she thought. Then she had an idea. She could dry the money in her microwave oven. She put the money in the microwave and switched it on. Then she went out of the kitchen. When she came back, she saw a fire inside the oven. She opened the oven door and put out the fire, but the money was all burnt.

The next day Lillian took her burnt money to the bank. The bank clerk told her that if he could see the numbers on the notes, he could replace them with new ones. He looked carefully at the notes but he could only find numbers on a few of them. He gave Lillian £17.00.

## post-elementary level

1. Tell me what you can remember about the story.

2. How much money did Lillian win?

3. Why did the money get wet?

4. How did she try to dry it first of all?

5. What did she do next?

6. Was this a good idea?

7. Why did the bank not give Lillian all her money back?

8. How do you think Lillian was feeling in the end?

Adapted from *More True Stories* by Sandra Heyer, Copyright © 1990 ISBN 0 8013 0223 4. Reprinted by permission of Addison Wesley Longman

# Allen is a little disaster

Allen Davies is only five, but he has already had so many accidents. The youngster has cracked his head falling into an empty swimming pool, has chopped off the end of his finger with a penknife and has made himself ill by drinking half a bottle of Dettol.

Each time another disaster strikes, Allen is taken to the Children's Hospital in Sydenham. He is such a regular visitor to the hospital that he thinks that one of the nurses is his sister! Now Allen's father is so grateful that he has raised £6,500 for the hospital to buy a monitor to measure babies' breathing and temperature.

Allen's mother Margaret said, "It all started when Allen was a year old. He fell over and cut himself and had to have stitches in his forehead. Since then he hasn't stopped. He has been taken to hospital at least ten times. The latest accident happened when he climbed onto a shelf and managed to open his father's penknife. He chopped the end of his finger off and had to have it sewn back on."

A nurse at the hospital said, "Whenever we see Allen coming in again, we all shout "What have you been doing this time?" Allen's older brothers have also had their share of accidents and have all been treated at Sydenham. Robert, aged 15, broke his ankle, and Lee, 13, injured his neck while riding a motorbike.

## intermediate level

1.   Tell me in your own words what this story is about.

2.   Can you remember some of the accidents Allen has had?

3.   Why does he think that the nurse is his sister?

4.   How has Allen's father helped at the hospital?

5.   When did Allen start having accidents?

6.   What happened to Allen's brothers?

7.   What do the nurses think about Allen?

Adapted from **John and Liz Soars**, *Headway Upper Intermediate* 1987 and reprinted by permission of Oxford University Press.

# Turkish Wedding

You must never miss a Turkish wedding! I was invited to a wedding which took place in a registry office at Kadikoy on the shore of the Bosphorus Sea. Before setting off to enjoy the day we dressed in our very best clothes. We drove first to the bride's home some miles outside the city and we waited for the groom to appear. Soon after all the guests had arrived outside the house, the young man appeared, to loud cheering and clapping from the crowd, in the wedding car - a limousine specially decked out with ribbons and a large doll, dressed as a bride in a white dress, attached to the bonnet. The groom then disappeared into the bride's house.

Minutes later the couple appeared, the groom dressed in a traditional black, formal suit with a flower, and the bride in a beautiful, European-style wedding dress with a long train and a veil. People cheered, some children threw confetti over the beaming couple as they made for their car. And then, with a roar, the bridal car disappeared at top speed! Everyone laughed as I found myself being pushed into another car and in no time we were off in pursuit of the groom. As we tore along the driver explained the reason for the rush:

"You see, if I can stop the groom's car, then he must pay me a fine in order to get past. If he can't pay the fine, he won't get to the registry office and he won't get married."

## Intermediate level

1. Tell me in your own words as much as you can about the story.

2. Which country does the wedding take place in?

3. Where did they go first?

4. How did the bridegroom get to the house?

5. What was on the front of the car?

6. What was the bride wearing?

7. Why was everyone laughing as the bridal car drove off?

Adapted from *In the Picture*, by Tricia Hedge, © 1985. ISBN 0 17 555396 3 Reprinted by permission of Addison Wesley Longman.

# Spelling Dictations

## Notes to accompany the spelling dictations

The spelling dictations are to be used to conduct an error analysis of the student's spelling strengths and weaknesses and approaches to spelling. For a detailed description of the analysis methodology, see *Diagnosing Dyslexia*.

The spelling passages have been specially produced to cover a range of sounds and spelling patterns in English, but with subject matter and vocabulary that should be relatively familiar to the students. They are based on similar passages devised by Margaret Peters[4]. They are all 100 words in length in order to give easy percentages.

The passages are graded in difficulty, Level 1 is for elementary learners, Level 2 is post-elementary, and Level 3 is for intermediate.. When selecting the level, tutors should bear in mind that they need from 20 - 25 errors in order to make an accurate assessment.

A student's spelling errors may be due to her using strategies from her first language, rather than to visual or auditory processing difficulties. For instance, if she speaks a language like Chinese, she may have difficulty in sounding out at all. If she speaks a phonetically regular language like Spanish, she may spell phonetically. Use the information you have gained about the student's own language(s) to help your assessment of her spelling.

You will also need to take into account the amount and type of instruction she has had about spelling in English when making the assessment.

## *Diagnostic Dictation (Level 1)*

My daughter was there, waiting for me at the airport gate. She was married now and her husband had a good job in the Post Office. She had no children yet so she still looked fresh and young, not like me.

We took the airport bus into the busy city centre. It was expensive, but it felt special. Then we got another bus to her home.

The house she lived in was nice but cold. The neighbours on both sides were not English. I always thought England was only for the English. Now I know better and I like it.

## Diagnostic Dictation (Level 2)

When father brought my mother and elder brother to Britain, before I was born, he reckoned it was unnecessary for mum to learn English. He thought he, my brother, and later my sister and I would always manage in emergencies.

One day, while everyone was out except mum, a pan in the kitchen caught fire. We returned to find the fire brigade and lots of smoke and dirty water. We all wondered how mum managed to call the emergency services, as she did not speak English.

Later she told us about the English class she had been attending in secret.

## Diagnostic Dictation (Level 3)

Every day immigrants and refugees have difficulty with government departments. Recently an acquaintance of mine, married with three children in this country, attracted the scrutiny of the Social Security authorities because they did not believe he was conscientious about seeking work. He scarcely speaks English, and is unaware of the regulations relating to the national benefit system, but the officials who interviewed and assessed him seemed completely unsympathetic to his plight and ordered him to enrol on an English course.

All the courses in his borough were full, but he was forbidden to search elsewhere. He is still experiencing frustration.

# Diagnostic Reports

The following reports give examples of the kind of things to include when diagnosing bilingual dyslexic students. The section starts with a comparison between reports of two students from Somalia, one who is dyslexic and one who is not. This has been included in order to demonstrate the differences between features of dyslexia and factors due largely to cultural and educational background. Then reports of a Moroccan student, and a Bengali student are given. Finally, there is an example of guidance notes for independent study given to the Bengali student when he stopped receiving additional support.

## A comparison of two students

Halima and Zainab (not their real names) were referred for dyslexia assessment. Both were from Somalia, both had spent most of their childhood fleeing from the Civil War. Both had spent only six months in school in Somalia. Both had attended the same secondary school in South London, Halima for 4 years and Zainab for 3 years before coming to College. Both were in their first year of an ESOL Foundation course. Halima was dyslexic, Zainab was not. What was the difference?

**Halima displayed a wide discrepancy between oral and writing abilities.** After four years in England, she spoke fluent English, with a slight London accent, and responded fully to English interview questions asked at normal speed. However her reading and writing were at the level expected of a 6 year old child in infant school.

**Zainab's literacy skills, though poorer than her oral ones, were near enough not to be remarkable.** She was not as fluent as Halima in speaking, her knowledge of vocabulary was not as wide, and she needed interview questions to be spoken at a slower speed. But her reading and writing were of a higher level at approximately the level expected of a 9 or 10 year old.

**Halima was unable to discriminate sounds and relate sounds to letters.** She could not break down words phonetically, or hear rhyme. When she read to me, she relied heavily on context and had no strategies for decoding unfamiliar words. She was unable to read simple one syllable 'non' words, again indicating that she could not relate sounds to letters. Her writing ability was far below her proficiency in spoken English. She took ten minutes to write about four very simple sentences. Her spelling was erratic - the was spelt correctly and incorrectly in the same passage. She spelt Somalia wrong; this was a word she must have been required to write hundreds of times in her four years in London. Other spellings were bizarre - *taehtr* for *teacher, beteew* for *behind, fani* for *frightened*.

Dyslexia and the Bilingual Learner; *Assessing and Teaching Adults and Young People who Speak English as an Additional Language*

43

**Zainab used phonic strategies to sound out words she did not recognise when she read.** These were almost all new words to her, ones that she did not know how to say and did not understand, and so it was reasonable to expect her to have difficulty in reading them. Her spelling was almost correct, and was based on phonologically accurate and visually reasonable guesses. For instance, she spelt *Vietnam*, a word she would not have learnt, as *Vetname*.

**Halima did not respond, even when given extra tuition.** At school she had attended extra language support sessions twice a week and was being taught basic literacy skills, including phonics, at college. In spite of this, she still found it impossible to relate sounds to letters.

**Zainab improved very quickly.** She learnt her spellings easily, and still remembered them at the end of term. Her reading improved dramatically as her knowledge of English vocabulary increased.

**Halima had other indicators for dyslexia** including confusion between left and right, an inability to remember facts (including her own telephone number), problems with copying from the board, and sequencing difficulties.

**Zainab had no other indicators for dyslexia.** Her memory was good, she had no left/right confusion, or difficulties in sequencing.

# Report on B.

## Background

B is from Morocco and came to Britain at the age of 22. His first language is Arabic and he was largely educated in French which he started at the age of 8. At primary school, he was a little slow at learning to read but he had considerable problems with writing, particularly in Arabic as several of his brothers and father had too. Although his problems were recognised by the school, he was able to concentrate on Maths and Science which he was very good at. In class he is a very able student and there is a marked discrepancy between his oral performance and his written one.

He shows some evidence of language disorder in that he has to make considerable effort to concentrate when listening and is easily distracted by background noise. In addition, he has some difficulty in pronouncing multisyllabic words and retrieving words in all three languages.

He also has difficulties remembering the alphabet and months in the right order, gets left and right confused and can get lost easily, all common among students with dyslexia. This may be linked to mixed laterality in that he is right-handed and left-eyed. However, his visual short term memory is good, particularly for numbers and calculations.

## Reading

B does not enjoy reading and therefore does not do it for pleasure. In a Reading Miscue Analysis he read a moderately difficult text quite fluently but with several mistakes. These were due to B not recognising the word and being only partially successful at sounding out words, for instance *'bigs"* for *"peaks"* *"sexful"* for *"successful"*. He sometimes left off the end of the word, for instance *"gradual"* for *"gradualness"*. His comprehension was poor on details except number facts which he remembered well, but he understood the main idea of the text.

## Spelling

In a spelling dictation, B got 53% of the words wrong. Of these, 60% were due to sounds misheard or omitted,. for instance *"sedent"* for *"southern"* *"resetely"* for *"recently"*. Forty percent were spelt as they sounded without an awareness of spelling conventions, for instance *"prisition"* for *"precision,"* *"surfese"* for *"surface."*

## Writing

B has an awkward style with many letters poorly formed. He claims his handwriting in both French (the language of most of his education and the same

---

script as English) and Arabic is equally bad. His grasp of grammar and punctuation is incomplete.

## Conclusion

B has specific learning difficulties (dyslexia) predominantly of an auditory processing nature.

## Recommendations for HE

1.  B should work systematically on words, particularly by breaking words up into meaningful parts. Meaning of suffixes may be helpful. He needs to learn words in groups of similar spelling to internalise spelling conventions. A multisensory method, with an emphasis on visual strategies and words within words, may help him remember.

2.  B would benefit from acquiring word-processing skills and should be encouraged to acquire a PC with a word processing function, plus a spell check. This would offset the difficulty in reading his writing and help correct his spellings. It may be useful for him to do any long written component of an exam on a word processor.

3.  In addition, the programme "Thinksheet" would be a help to B in organising written work.

4.  B would benefit from specialist support at university.


*Ann Butterfield (Dyslexia Support Tutor)*

# M. R.

## Background

M. is from Bangladesh. He came to this country when he was five. At the age of nine he went back to Bangladesh for a year, and attended school there for some of that time. When he returned to London there were no other Asians in his class. He was told off because he couldn't understand, so he started to misbehave. At secondary school he mixed with "*a lot of naughty children*". He sometimes found it hard to concentrate, and thus found the work boring, and so misbehaved again. Now he is keen to learn to read and write better.

Since childhood, M. has had a lot of problems with his ears. He has been told he may need an operation, but has never actually had one. He listens, but sometimes he cannot take in what he hears. He finds that some days are better than others.

## Language

History M. speaks Sylheti with his father, and English with his brothers. He never learnt to read and write standard Bengali which is different from Sylheti. His brothers can all read and write English and Bengali. M. is the only one who finds reading and writing difficult.

M. speaks London English fluently, and his comprehension is good. He had no difficulty at all either understanding or replying to the interview questions, and these were asked at normal speed.

## Reading

M.'s reading is halting, even with a basic level text. He has a lot of difficulties with texts at a post-basic level. He has good strategies relating to context and meaning, and can guess, but not always accurately (for instance reading *London* for *England* in a text about immigration). He can use the initial sounds with the context to guess an unknown word, but does not appear to be able to use phonics after the initial sound (for instance reading *interest* for *introduce*).

His comprehension of the basic level texts is good, he was able to recall and re-tell the story and answer comprehension questions. At funny stories, he laughed in the right places.

He was unable to read nine out of ten simple 'non-words'.

He enjoys reading, and regularly borrowed my books to take home and read.

## Spelling and dictation

M.'s spelling shows lack of awareness of common spelling patterns and possible visual processing problems. For instance he wrote *mane* for *many*, *bezze* for *busy*. He also reverses letters, for instance *poeple* for *people*, *fuor* for *four*, *tary* for *try*, *pals* for *place*. The last two could be explained by the fact that in Sylheti there are no consonant clusters, thus he inserts a vowel sound, as he would if he said the word. There are also signs of auditory discrimination difficulties - for instance *brokes* for *bricks*, *lanleg* for *language*, *fatma* for *Vietnam*, *soct* for *store*. Also possible motor difficulties, for instance telescoping - *rumber* for *remember*.

He spells words inconsistently; sometimes they are right, other times near, other times quite unlike the correct spelling.

In dictation, he often omits a word - he cannot even begin to try and spell it.

## Writing

His handwriting is small and would be quite neat except for crossings out and over-writing where he thinks he may have made a mistake. He does not join up his handwriting. He does not reverse letters.

His composition is basic, his written vocabulary and organisation of ideas much less sophisticated than his spoken English.

His use of punctuation is erratic, he appears to pepper his text with full stops and capital letters, but they have little relationship with the organisation of the text.

## Other indicators for Dyslexia

M. finds concentration difficult - for instance he got distracted halfway through the diagnostic interview. He has identified this as a problem, at college and before at school. He finds that some days it is better than others.

He is left-handed, and holds his pen awkwardly.

He liked maths, but found learning his times tables very difficult. He finds long numbers difficult. His brother eventually taught him to tell the time, but this was quite late, when he was about 10 or 11 years old.

He cannot remember the months in the right order - he knows them, but does not know which comes first, or how they follow on from each other. He writes down telephone numbers as he can remember them only occasionally.

## Conclusions

In spite of his disrupted education and the fact that he is learning in his second language, M.'s reading and writing difficulties appear greater than would be normally expected. These are due to dyslexia, mainly of an auditory perceptual nature.

In the light of these difficulties, I would recommend that M. be given extra individual help with reading and writing, placing particular emphasis on visual approaches to learning spellings, as well as strategies for greater accuracy in reading. He should be put on an individual spelling programme which should also help his reading. He should also be encouraged to develop cursive writing, which will help his spelling. He needs to understand and use simple punctuation, both in reading and in writing.

Tutors should be made aware that M's difficulties are due to dyslexia, so that he is not dismissed as lazy or unmotivated.

*Helen Sunderland*

# M. - Notes for self-study, following the end of extra support tuition

## General

You find it hard to discriminate sounds, and this makes it difficult for you to 'sound out' words when you read and spell. This may have origins in the hearing problems that you had as a child. This means that you have to work particularly hard at remembering what words **look** like, as you can't always hear what they **sound** like.

Here are a few ideas for you.

## Spelling

You know how to do this now.

- Choose the words you want to spell,

- Find some others with the same pattern (this is so you become familiar with what English spelling patterns look like). Highlight the pattern.

- Do the Look, Cover, Write, Check routine with them **every day.** Unless you do them every day, you will not remember them in the long term, though you may remember them for a few days.

- After a week, get someone (your friend or someone in your family) to test you.

- Write each word in a sentence, so you get used to using it.

- Don't try and learn more than 6 or 7 new words a week, or you will forget them more quickly.

## Reading

Your reading is quite good. You obviously enjoy reading, and you should keep on with it.

- Try and read for pleasure for at least half an hour per day. This can be magazines, newspapers, story and fact books - whatever you are interested in.

- Take books out of the college library. Join the public library - you will find lots more books there.

- If you do not know what a word is, don't just guess, try and work it out from the sound of the first letters. Ask someone to check if you have it right. If you do this, you will continue to build up the number of words that you can recognise by sight.

## Writing

You need to get more used to the sound of written English, which is very different from spoken English.

One way to do this is to listen to books being read.

- Reading books yourself will help.

- Borrow 'spoken word' tapes of books - the college library may have some, and your local public library definitely should, though you may need to pay a small amount of money to borrow them. Listen to the books being read. This will make you familiar with how written English is put together.

- Practise writing 'joined up' - this will help your spelling.

- Do lots of writing - keep a diary, write to friends - try and use the new words you have learnt to spell and to read.

### Good luck!

# Guidelines for ESOL and Language Support Teachers

## A. The dyslexic learning style

Dyslexia may be usefully viewed as a difference in learning style.

As the processing weaknesses of dyslexic learners are primarily to do with language and sequence which belong to the specialisation of the left hemisphere of the brain, their cognitive strengths, whether through compensation or superior development, are often in right hemispheric specialisations. These include visualising (in terms of imagery), spatial ability, and a tendency to look for inter-relationships as opposed to sequential or temporal ones (such as cause and effect). Right hemisphere specialisations also include non-linguistic aspects of language such as mood, tone, humour, emotion.

In addition, because dyslexic students have difficulties coding language to store and retrieve linguistic information, they tend to rely on semantic coding, that is, meaning and associations, rather than faulty auditory and/or visual memory. Short-term memory relies significantly on phonological coding, (we repeat or rehearse information in order to remember it), and it also relies on visual memory for letter patterns and word recognition; these are areas where dyslexic people are weak.

By not emphasising rote verbal learning but rather helping dyslexic students to make use of personal associations and meaningful connections to remember, learning can be significantly improved.

By helping them to picture, or get an image of a situation, rather than trying to remember a sequence, again learning will be more effective.

Dyslexic people are also often concrete learners; rather than learn from the generalisation and apply it, they are more likely to learn through 'hands-on' experience and make generalisations later. It is easy as a teacher to forget the abstract nature of written language particularly, for instance the arbitrary relationships of letters to sounds. It is often easier for a dyslexic person to see a connection between letter or sentence patterns by moving them around physically (as in plastic letters) than by trying to see the connection on a page of printed text.

Research has shown that much of the normal language class - or indeed any class - is auditory: the teacher and students talking. For those with auditory processing difficulties, such extended concentration, especially when new material is being presented and even more especially when it is in an additional language, can be very tiring and easily result in 'tuning out'.

Dyslexia and the Bilingual Learner; *Assessing and Teaching Adults and Young People who Speak English as an Additional Language*

53

The more aware the teacher is of the individual learner's strengths and weaknesses, the easier it is to avoid approaches which will repeat past failure and to find approaches more likely to be successful.

Perceptual learning preferences can be especially helpful in finding strategies for language learning. Most students, not only dyslexic ones, will find they have a learning preference which may be either auditory, visual or kinaesthetic. Multisensory approaches can enable students to identify their preferred learning style and this in turn creates more confidence about learning and more autonomy in finding successful learning strategies.

For a fuller discussion of the dyslexic learning style and its implications for teaching, see *Demystifying Dyslexia* (details in **Useful Books and Resources**).

The following approaches should benefit everyone, whether or not they are dyslexic. Using strategies that involve the whole brain, not just the left side, have been shown to improve learning for all students.

Though many of them may be approaches already commonly in use, we are emphasising those methods that will particularly help dyslexic learners who may have had their confidence undermined in the past by the use of approaches that were inappropriate for them.

They may involve re-thinking some of the 'sacred cows' of ESOL teaching; it is important to 'step back', forget all the "you must never......." and see what works for the individual student. Tutors need to be aware of students' individual learning differences and find ways to use their strengths to improve learning.

## B. Approaches to teaching

### 1. Use a multi-sensory approach

A multi-sensory approach works, not only because it is holistic, but because, for people with specific difficulties such as poor auditory or visual memories, it gives them more than one route to learning.

Tutors can combine approaches from all of the following ones.

### Visual Approaches

Use images - for presentation, in drills, on worksheets and on reference sheets. Even if students can read quite well, it will help to jog the memory and make connections.

Encourage the development of images to aid comprehension and memory. For instance, if students are reading, get them to try and visualise the scene.

Use wall posters with graphics and words to reinforce work done in the class. Put them just above eye level.

Use colour - on the board and on materials where possible. Get students to use colour too - to highlight (for instance 'ed' endings) or to circle key points, vocabulary, parts of language patterns etc. For instance, if showing a language pattern on the board;

Eritrea is hot

Eritrea is hotter than England

England is cold

England is colder than Eritrea

the stem (hot, cold) and the ending (er) could be in red and blue respectively. Use colours to highlight the use of particular tenses - for instance red for the simple past, yellow for the present perfect, green for the simple present.

To teach language patterns, have blocks of sentences on different coloured cards, for instance

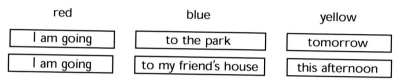

let students put them together.

Label objects, so that students associate the word with the object. Students could do this as a learning activity, labelling the object, and then as a listening activity, removing certain labels.

## Sound:

Use music, songs and chants for presentation, practising language patterns or extending vocabulary. (see *Jazz Chants, English Through Song* for ideas of how to do this.) Then when students wish to recall particular structures or vocabulary, they will have the music to help them remember. Get students to beat out rhythms for spelling as well as for pronunciation, for instance click fingers or clap on the double letters as they spell *bigger* - *b i gg*(clap twice) *e r.*

## Kinaesthetic/whole body approach:

Use movements as a memory jogger (as in the song *'head and shoulders, knees and toes'*), trace words for spelling or handwriting, use whole arm movements (i.e. tracing the word in the air) for people who have difficulty with writing the script. Let students use plastic letters to make words and reinforce spelling patterns (they can use plastic letters that have vowels in a different colour).

This approach also includes drama - students can act out stories, rather than just reading or telling them, - and role play - these also help to make the context of language use clear. When you use mime or gestures (for instance pointing over your shoulder for the past tense or counting on fingers for the number of syllables in a word), get students to join in and use them too. Do the same

Dyslexia and the Bilingual Learner; *Assessing and Teaching Adults and Young People who Speak English as an Additional Language*

55

when beating out rhythms for pronunciation.

Ensure students get up and move around for some of the class. This also raises the energy level and helps concentration when students sit down again.

Reinforce learning by using more than one sense; for example, read a text and listen to the tape at the same time, act or use prompts (pictures or words) to stimulate speech or writing.

### 2. Use Variety

Change activities to reinforce the same language teaching point. Keep activities short (because of students' concentration span), but keep them related to the same teaching point for reinforcement and so they do not become overloaded.

### 3. Use a Holistic Approach

Let students see the whole picture first, for instance let them see the past, present and future tenses together, before taking one and concentrating on teaching it.

When reading, present the overview through discussion or listening to a tape first.

### 4. Use Inductive Methods

Most dyslexic learners are inductive thinkers - they go from the particular (lots of examples) to the general or rule, rather than the other way round. In ESOL, we often give the rule (for instance *"put **ed** on to the verb stem to make the past tense"*) and then go on to practise particular examples. Instead of doing this, let students work out the rule from the examples. *Self-Access worksheets, Volume 1*, has some good spelling exercises which do this, but it can also be done with grammar. (See *The Teacher's Video* for an example of teaching reported speech by this method).

### 5. Think about the 'Order of skills'

Re-think the traditional order of skills - i.e. listening, speaking, reading and writing. Be flexible about the variety of ways that students may learn. Different students may have different ways of acquiring skills depending on their strengths and weaknesses. For instance many dyslexic students learn to read through learning to spell and write. A student with auditory processing difficulties may find it difficult to listen and repeat a structure or language pattern, and may find it easier to write a phrase down (possibly transliterated into his own script) and read it back before trying to say it.

### 6. Strategies for Teaching Spelling

Spelling may need to be approached more systematically than is usual in an ESOL class; dyslexic students often have difficulties with spelling, but with the right strategies, they can really make progress. The list of **Useful Books and Resources** contains some excellent resources with detailed spelling approaches. Here are some general guidelines and strategies, useful for all students, whether dyslexic or not.

- contextualise spellings to be learnt, take them from student writing, rather than from a general list

- combine strategies that use a range of senses (see ideas below)

- review regularly with 'little and often' practice

- encourage students to use the strategies that work best for them. For example, some students with weak auditory memories (that is, difficulty processing sounds) will prefer visual strategies and vice versa.

- **praise** the students for what they have got right! For example the spelling 'freind' has the beginning and ending correct - it just has an error in the middle.

# Strategies

## Auditory: *use your ears and your voice*

- split word into sections , spell aloud in a rhythm:   *n-e-c e-s-s a-r-y.* Click or tap fingers on the *c* and *ss* at the same time

- split double letters and say the word aloud in sections: ac/com/mod/ation to help hear and remember the 2m's and c's

- exaggerate the sounds, or split words up in an unusual way to hear the bits that are usually 'swallowed' for instance, *Feb/ru/ary* ( though take care to practise the correct pronunciation as well!)

## Visual: **use your eyes**

- highlight the problem area of a word using different colour, highlighter, bold on computer, for instance lib**rar**y. ( **Avoid** writing part of the word in upper case for emphasis (libRARy) which can cause confusion).

- look for a familiar small word inside the longer one, for instance student who writes 'becase' can look for 'use' (beca**use**). Highlight the small word and ' say it funny' if it helps. Get the student to combine the two words in a sentence, saying and writing them, highlighting the 'use', for instance 'I **use** my pen beca**use** I want to write.'

- highlight common letter patterns, for instance r **ain**, tr **ain** etc. Dyslexic students often have difficulty **hearing** rhyme, but this works well as a visual strategy

Dyslexia and the Bilingual Learner; *Assessing and Teaching Adults and Young People who Speak English as an Additional Language*

57

- draw a box round the word to visualise its length and shape

- find distinctive visual patterns and break up words accordingly, for instance acc **ommo** dation, r **ece** ive

## Kinaesthetic: use your body

Spelling is partly a motor skill, so these strategies will help get the automatic flow of the word going

- start by getting the student to join two or three letters in letter strings, for instance *ing, ain*

- get the student to trace the word with her finger on the table, without lifting off mid-word. Get her to trace the word in the air and spell aloud at the same time.

- help students to practise a cursive script: this helps automatic flow and stops the doubt creeping in every time the student lifts up the pen

- Typing can help, so that students can remember the word by the position of the letters on the keyboard.

## Spelling rules

- Disjointed abstract rules are unlikely to help, but students may enjoy working out the rule from examples

- Students may need spelling conventions made explicit for instance that 'ph' sounds like 'f', or that 'q' is always followed by 'u'. They can be familiarised with likely word endings, for instance the 'ee' sound on the end of a word is usually spelt with a 'y' (as in *happy*.)

## Practice makes perfect

Regular, little and often, daily practice will work far better than writing the word many times over at one time, which only holds the word in the short term memory. Regular review will aid the motor memory and help the word to get into the long term memory store. This practice needs to be complemented by the above spelling strategies, suited to individual learning preferences, which will aid recall.

The **LOOK, COVER, WRITE, CHECK** system is described fully in the recommended spelling books, but here is a brief summary:

- divide a sheet into columns, one for each day

- write the words to be practised down the left hand side (if students do this themselves, be sure to check their spelling)

- each day, students look at each word, recall the strategy they are using to remember it, cover up the word and write it from memory, saying the word aloud as they write

- they then check the word back carefully letter by letter. (This can be quite hard at first; show the student how to follow the two words along in parallel, by tracking with the finger and a pen.)

- if the word is wrong, they write the whole word again, to get the motor memory of the feel of the letters in sequence

- if it is correct, leave it till the next day

- at the end of a week test the student on the words; the next week get students to write them in short sentences.

## 7.   Strategies for Teaching Phonics

It is very important to give people access to the sound/symbol relationship and phonics should be taught in a systematic way. Students also need to know the names of letters as well as the sounds they are associated with. They may need to be taught common blends, - *sh, ch, th* etc. in an explicit way. When teaching phonics it has been shown to be more successful to teach connected groups of sound, such as *b - ed* and *r - ed* rather than *b - e - d* and *r - e - d*. This can progress to *be - d* and *re - d*. However, it is important to remember that some people will find phonics difficult and may not be able to distinguish certain sounds. They will need to concentrate on visual strategies.

## 8.   Accessing reading and listening material

Put the passage into context through pre-task activities such as discussion or pictures. Listen and read together, then read or listen with a task. Encourage them to picture the scene while they listen. Do not expect students to remember what they have heard if they have not been given a task to do. For instance, instead of saying, "*Listen to this tape*" and then afterwards ask, "*What did she say?*" say something like, "*Listen to this tape of a phone call. Pick out where and when the two speakers arrange to meet*".

# C.   Some general points

It is said that dyslexic learners are quick forgetters rather than slow learners. You may be disappointed at how little a student has retained from one lesson to the next. There is a need for constant repetition, reinforcement and review within each session as well as between sessions.

Dyslexic students learn better if they understand the reason for the activity. You need to be explicit about **why** as well as **how** you expect them to do something. (We realise this is not always possible with less fluent students, though more advanced students can sometimes be used to translate.)

Encourage students to be aware of their own strengths, strategies and learning styles. Get them to tape themselves speaking and reading and to analyse their performance.

Students learn better if the whole brain is involved in the process. This means including emotional as well as cognitive activities. For instance, ask students to shut their eyes and think of a beautiful place, or start the class with some happy music. Reminiscence activities also involve this part of the brain.

Dyslexic students are concrete learners; they need particularly personalised strategies to learn effectively. Before any activity - drilling, reading, listening, - ensure that the context is very clear, and personalise it to the experience of the students if possible; for instance in map-reading activities use a map of the local area rather than one from a text book. Avoid the kind of de-contextualised grammar practice sentences that are common in many grammar text books. Such activities are very difficult for them to learn from. Instead, you can use inductive methods (see above), produce practice sentences from the context you have already used to present the language (for instance from a story or dialogue), or get students to produce their own practice sentences.

## D.    ESOL teaching techniques that could cause difficulty

**Copying from the board** can be difficult, because it means holding the words in the short term memory before transferring them to paper. Think about other ways information can be conveyed, (for instance handouts) or allow plenty of time and check the accuracy of what students have copied. You may need to indicate to students what is important to write down, though it is true that students usually want to copy everything, which is another reason to limit what is written. It is particularly important to write clearly on the board.

When teaching particular words or structures, try to encourage students to develop their visual memory by looking at the board, visualising the words in their 'minds eye' and writing without looking, instead of copying. You can rub words out and then put them back in for students to check whether they have written them correctly.

**Substitution tables**, particularly on the board, can cause difficulties for students, because of visual tracking. That is, they find it difficult to go up and down the columns, keep information in their heads, and then transfer this information into a sentence along a straight line. Instead of substitution tables, show patterns:

| Angola | is | in | Africa |
|---|---|---|---|
| England | is | in | Europe |
| India | is | in | Asia |
| Angola and Zaire | are | in | Africa |
| England and Spain | are | in | Europe |
| India and Iran | are | in | Asia |

preferably with *is* and *are* highlighted in different colours.

**Drills** - dyslexic learners have difficulties in holding information in their short term memory. If they have a poor auditory memory, this can make oral drills very difficult.

When drilling, don't have too many variables, use pictures or props as memory joggers, and make sure the student understands the context of the drill. Use music, rhythm and songs to aid the auditory memory.

Let students write down the drill and read it if this helps them to learn the drill, but make sure they also practise it without reading (eventually).

Dyslexia and the Bilingual Learner;  *Assessing and Teaching Adults and Young People who Speak English as an Additional Language*

61

# Guidelines for Dyslexia Support Teachers

The following issues have already been mentioned in **Cultural and Linguistic Factors that may Affect Diagnosis**, and readers may like to refer back to that Section before reading this one. However, in this Section the issues are approached from the perspective of supporting and teaching students rather than diagnosing their dyslexia. As well as discussing the issues that will influence their learning, this Section suggests strategies and resources to use when teaching bilingual dyslexic learners.

## 1. Cultural issues

Unfamiliar cultural contexts can affect how much a student understands of a reading passage. This can be true of fiction and vocational materials.

For example, a student on a further education business studies course was asked to read some promotional material for hot breakfast cereals. This talked about how popular the cereals were in Scotland. The student did not know that Scotland is in the north, that it is colder than England, or that there is a tradition of eating hot porridge in Scotland. Thus, though she could understand every word of the reading passage, the point of it was lost on her because she was not familiar with the cultural context. She was bewildered by the whole thing.

Similarly, students in higher education were asked to compare the National Curriculum Orders concerning bilingualism for Wales and for England. A recently arrived student, who spoke and read English fluently, found the task impossible until a fellow student explained what the National Curriculum was, and that bilingualism in Wales was about Welsh and English, whereas bilingualism in England concerned English and migrant/refugee languages. Again, the student could read and understand every word, but was mystified by the overall task, because she did not understand the cultural context.

Support tutors need to ensure that their students are familiar with the cultural context and explicit and implicit cultural references that may affect their understanding of any reading they have to do. If choosing texts for extra reading practice, these also need to be culturally appropriate. What is understood, and what is appropriate, will depend on the individual student, and so tutors will need to discuss these issues with their students.

## 2. Influence of other languages.

Features from students' other language(s) can affect how they learn to read and write English. This can affect learning spelling, handwriting, grammar and organisation of sentences and longer texts (see **Cultural and Linguistic**

**Factors that may affect Diagnosis.**)

For instance, as spelling is phonetically regular in Spanish, Spanish speaking students may expect it to be the same in English. As Chinese does not express the past tense through changed verb endings, Chinese students may forget to add 'ed' to make the past.

Tutors and students can learn together, if these issues are discussed during support sessions. Both will begin to understand why students may be making mistakes, and students can learn to watch out for potential difficulties.

*Self Access Grammar* (see **Useful Books and Resources**) has some useful worksheets which could be a starting point for the discussion. *Learner English* (see **Useful Books and Resources**) gives a narrative comparison of many world languages with English.

Tutors may also find it useful to talk to other tutors, particularly of ESOL or languages. They may be able to give information about the characteristics of particular languages, or the difficulties that students speaking particular languages may commonly have in learning English.

## 3.  Difficulties in other languages

Students can give tutors information about difficulties they have had in reading and writing in their languages. If this discussion is part of the support, then it can help both tutors and students identify where problems may recur, or where problems are more likely to be due to learning a new language. For instance, if a student always had neat handwriting in Arabic, it is likely that poor English handwriting is due to the difference in script, and will improve with practice. If, however, she was always a messy and slow writer, even after years of schooling in Sudan, then it is possible that she has motor processing difficulties, and will have to work very hard to improve her English handwriting.

## 4.  English Language Development

Bilingual students may need to develop their spoken English in order to improve their literacy. Vocabulary extension exercises, listening practice and oral work may all be useful. In order to help learners retain new vocabulary tutors can encourage them to relate it to vocabulary in their own language, as well as vocabulary extension through word association games and discussion. The student can make a dictionary with translations in her own language of the words she learns. It is important to ensure that the student actually knows, understands and can say any word that she is being asked to learn as part of the spelling programme.

Listening can be taught in much the same way as reading, by using directed activities related to the listening passage. For instance, students can be asked to listen out for particular words (linking with vocabulary development), for what the piece is about (the gist), for the main points, for inferred meanings.

Dyslexia and the Bilingual Learner;  *Assessing and Teaching Adults and Young People who Speak English as an Additional Language*

*63*

Information from the piece can be transferred into writing, onto a table or in a cloze passage. Links can be made between reading skills and listening skills. Students can be shown that, just as there is no need to understand every word when listening in order to get the main points, the same applies when reading. However, if they wish to understand everything, then they may need to read or listen several times.

Some English language teaching tapes and books are included in the bibliography, but tutors could work with tapes from the radio, relating to the students' vocational or academic area, or with tapes the students have made of their lectures.

Work on pronunciation may help with spelling. If students are having difficulty making or hearing sounds, it may be that the sound does not exist in their languages. Tutors can discuss this with them and ask them to think of the nearest sound in their language(s). Techniques such as exaggerated pronunciation may help. Here the tutor exaggerates the sound and mouth position - for instance lengthening the already long vowel in *Sheeeeep*, and stretching the lips to the side of the face. The student looks at the position of the mouth, tongue, and lips, and then tries herself, possibly using a mirror. *Ship and Sheep* (see **Useful Books and Resources)** shows the mouth position for the sounds of British English.

## 5. Technology

Use technology where it may be able to help.

For instance, students can tape themselves speaking and analyse the tape for errors, thus becoming more aware of grammatical and phonological difficulties they may have. (*Self Access Grammar* has good examples of how students can start to categorise and learn from their grammatical mistakes.) They can use taped books or CD ROM with sound to hear how to pronounce the words they are reading.

## 6. Register and text conventions

Students who have had much of their education overseas may have been taught different text conventions - for instance they may be required to be more formal. In many countries the written word is revered, and therefore many learners have a dislike of colloquial language. Teachers emphasising shortened forms and colloquialisms may meet strong resistance from students who come from this tradition. Students sometimes use what may be considered by our conventions to be 'flowery' language. Tutors often feel uneasy about challenging students' style, but if it is looked at as a difference in conventions, and the two conventions compared, then the student can choose to change his style when he is writing English and keep his old style when writing his language, if he so wishes.

On the other hand, there may be students who have had most of their education here but who do not speak English except at school who thus may not know the more formal registers, for instance *purchase* for *buy*. Though, superficially, they seem fluent in English, they may in fact need help with academic or formal vocabulary and expressions, both in reading and writing.

As has already been mentioned in **Cultural and Linguistic Factors that may Affect Diagnosis,** other cultures may organise their ideas differently, both in speech and in writing. We tend to make our main point (as for instance in the topic sentence of a paragraph) and then go on to elaborate. In other cultures, for instance many of the Asian cultures, it is more common to end with the main point. Tutors need to discuss this with their students and be as explicit as possible about the organisation of the particular genre the student is trying to write, comparing it with how it would be written in the student's country.

Finally, layout conventions differ from country to country. Something as simple as how a letter is laid out can vary enormously and needs to be discussed, with conventions compared in the different countries.

## 7. Proof-reading

Students who have had most of their education overseas may not have been used to proof-reading their own work. In more formal systems, the teacher marks the work, corrects it, gives it back, and the student copies it out again, with the mistakes corrected. Students from this kind of education system may not understand the reasons for proof-reading, may think it is the job of the teacher, and may need to have a lot of discussion and explanation given before they feel comfortable with doing their own proof-reading.

## 8. Teaching Methods

Differences in teaching methods can cause difficulty for students who may not be sure what is expected of them at each stage of the class.

One student complained that she had not been given information she needed for an assignment. When the support tutor asked the class tutor about this, she was told that it was not true - the students had discussed the subject of the assignment in groups. However, the student, not used to group discussion as a teaching method, had not paid too much attention to the group discussion and had not taken notes. In effect, she was waiting for the 'real teaching' to begin. Support tutors can help by discussing teaching methods and expectations with their students, and by helping the students be clear about what they should do (that is, take notes) in different stages of the lesson. *The GNVQ Induction Pack* (see **Useful Books and Resources**) contains activities and materials that look at teaching and assessment methods, and allow students to draw on their experience of education in other parts of the world and relate it to education in this country.

Dyslexia and the Bilingual Learner;   *Assessing and Teaching Adults and Young People who Speak English as an Additional Language*

# Useful Books and Resources

## General Books on Dyslexia

**Adult Students and Dyslexia**  (1995) V. Goodwin and B. Thomson, Open University Press (includes audio cassette).

**Demystifying Dyslexia**, (1995), Marysia Krupska and Cynthia Klein,  London Language and Literacy Unit.

**Diagnosing Dyslexia**, (1993), Cynthia Klein, Basic Skills Agency.

**Dyslexia at College**, (1986)  T. Miles and D. Gilroy,

**Dyslexia, Signposts to Success**, a guide for dyslexic adults, (1995), compiled by Jo Matty, British Dyslexia Association.

**How to Detect and Manage Dyslexia**, (1997) Philomena Ott, Heinemann.

## Dyslexia and Language Learning

**Learning a Foreign Language:  Challenges for Students with Language Learning Difficulties,** (1995) Leonore Ganschow and Richard Sparks,  in *Dyslexia* Volume 1.

**Teaching Modern Languages to Pupils with Specific Learning Difficulties (Dyslexia)**, (1995), Tameside Metropolitan Borough Council, LDSS Support Service.

## Books about how languages work

**Learner English  A Teacher's Guide to Interference and Other Problems**. (9th edition 1995) Edited by M. Swan & B. Smith,  Cambridge University Press.

**Lessons from the Vietnamese** (for information on Vietnamese language), (1981 & out of print) by F. De La Motte, H Fraser, M Greatbanks, S Rees and A Slater, NEC.

**Ship or Sheep?** (1981) Ann Baker, Cambridge University Press (for information on the mouth position for pronunciation of English sounds)

**Sounds English** (1989) C. Fletcher and O'Connor, Longman.  (for information on pronunciation differences of students who speak other languages)

## For Diagnosis

**Use Your Eyes,** (2nd Edition  1992), Brown and Brown.

Dyslexia and the Bilingual Learner;    *Assessing and Teaching Adults and Young People who Speak English as an Additional Language*

*67*

### ESOL Teaching books:

**English through Song** (1996) Judith Silver, Silversong Publications.

**Jazz Chants**, (1978) Carolyn Graham, Oxford University Press.

**Self Access Worksheets 1** (1986) Erica Buckmaster, NEC.

**Self-Access Grammar (**1990) Erica Buckmaster, NEC.

**English Experience** materials, developed by an organisation with a 'brain friendly' approach to learning, catalogue available from English Experience, 25 Julian Road, Folkestone CT19 5HW.

### General books on learning

**Accelerate Your Learning**, (1992), Colin Rose and Louise Goll, obtainable from Accelerated Learning Systems Ltd, 50 Aylesbury Road, Aston Clinton, Aylesbury, Bucks, HP22 5AH.

**Errors and Expectations** (1977) M. Shaughnessy, Open University Press.

**Get Ahead - Mind Map Your Way to Success** (1991) Vanda North and Tony Buzan, Oakdale Printing Co.

**GNVQ Induction Pack** (1996), GNVQ Working Party, London Language and Literacy Unit.

**Teaching for the Two-sided Mind**, a guide to right brain/left brain education, (1986), Linda Verlee Williams, Simon & Schuster.

**Use Your Head,** (1982), Tony Buzan, BBC Publications.

**Computers and Typography**, Rosemary Sassoon, Intellect Books

### Spelling

**Making Sense of Spelling**, (1986) Robin Millar and Cynthia Klein, SENJIT, Institute of Education, 30 Bedford Way, London W1.

**Unscrambling Spelling,** (1990) Robin Millar and Cynthia Klein, Hodder & Stoughton.

**A Speller's Companion**, (1987), Hugh and Margaret Brown, Brown and Brown.

### Handwriting

**Here's Handwriting,** edited by Lesley Henderson, Scottish Community Education Council, West Coates House, Haymarket Terrace, Edinburgh EH12 5LQ. (Aimed at adults, nicely presented.)

**The Acquisition of a Second Writing system**, (1995), Rosemary Sassoon, Intellect.

## On Video

**Dyslexia: Symptoms.** Obtainable from Alpha Training, Chorlton Park Centre, Mauldeth Road West, Manchester M21 2SL. Adult dyslexic students describing their personal experience of how dyslexia affects them in areas such as reading, spelling, memory and direction.

**Get Ahead - Short Cut to Straight As**, Buzan Centres Ltd., 37 Waterloo Road, Bournemouth BH9 1BD.

**The Teacher's Video, An ESOL Tutor Training Resource,** (1996) London Language & Literacy Unit. See *Level 3 - Teaching a Grammar Point,* for an example of an inductive approach to teaching grammar.

**Teaching Adult Literacy, Unit B:  Strategies for Teaching Spelling,** ILEA. Obtainable from Educational Medial Internation, 235 Imperial Drive, Rayners Lane, Harrow, Middlesex HA2 7HE. Shows both a class and a one to one approach.

Dyslexia and the Bilingual Learner;    *Assessing and Teaching Adults and Young People who Speak English as an Additional Language*

69

REFERENCES

# References

1 Vellutino, FR and Scanlon, DM (1987) *Phonological Coding, Phonological Awareness and Reading Ability* in *Merrill-Palmer Quarterly 33.*

2 Klein, Hannah (1985) The Assessment and Management of Some Persisting Language Difficulties in the Learning Disabled, in *Children's Written Language Difficulties*, Ed. Snowling, NFER-Nelson

3 Peer, L. (1996) *Dyslexia and bi/multilingualism: In a class of their own.* unpublished MA (SEN) thesis. The Manchester Metropolitan University, Didsbury School of Education.

4 Peters, Margaret & Smith, Brigid D., (1993) *Spelling in Context: Strategies for Teachers and Learners,* NFER Nelson.

70     Dyslexia and the Bilingual Learner;    *Assessing and Teaching Adults and Young People who Speak English as an Additional Language*